The Truth About Orthodontics

A Consumer's Guide To A Beautiful Smile

John W. Graham, DDS,MD

ISBN: 0615992722
ISBN-13: 978-0615992723

Library of Congress Control Number: 2014937012
Sugarhouse Publishing, Salt Lake City, UT

To my beautiful wife and wonderful children.

Contents

I've been taught by some of the best physicians and dentists in the world, and for them, I am grateful. However, I have been taught far more by the wonderful patients I've had the great honor of treating. And I couldn't have treated any of those patients without the best staff in the world. Thank you all.

Introduction

Braces are for kids. Braces take forever. Most people who get braces need teeth pulled. My kid needs an expander.

Lies.

Lies.

Lies.

OK, I shouldn't be so dramatic, but we've all heard these things, and why not believe them? *For heaven's sake,* you might say, *I've seen plenty of kids in braces; they always seem to have them on forever, and they've usually had teeth pulled.* And you're right: all of the experiences mentioned above can happen, do happen, and usually shouldn't happen.

Yet such happenings are all ancient history in the world of modern orthodontics.

We've believed these misconceptions about orthodontics for years, and my hope is to shed some light on the untruths and outright lies—all in an effort to enlighten parents of children who would benefit from orthodontics, as well as any adults who want more beautiful, confident smiles themselves. This isn't a textbook, nor is it an exhaustive treatise on the current state of orthodontics. Instead, since the practice of "straightening teeth" has evolved so much in recent years, virtually eliminating the need for tooth extraction, headgear, and palatal expanders, I would prefer to call this little book simply an introduction to the current, wonderful world of *Modern Orthodontic Smile Design.*

My hope in writing this is to give you basic information on cutting-edge orthodontic techniques so that you can ask the questions that matter when you find yourself in an orthodontist's or general dentist's office.

One

Perspective

I'm an orthodontist. I'm a dentist. I'm a physician. I'm a father with children in orthodontic treatment, I'm married to a pediatric dentist who had orthodontic treatment as a teen and an adult, and I've been an orthodontic patient myself twice.

What makes me different from many orthodontists is my unique perspective on the profession. I have been involved in the creation of patented orthodontic devices, have been on the orthodontic faculty at two universities, and serve as a contributing editor to one of our profession's peer-reviewed journals. I'm a consultant to many orthodontic and medical device companies, and I've served our national association as an advisor. Several large orthodontic companies have used my patients as cover models for their marketing materials, and I've had a patient on the cover of the *American Journal of Orthodontics and*

Dentofacial Orthopedics, our most esteemed peer-reviewed journal. Because of my background and experience, I've been invited to lecture to thousands of orthodontists and their staffs all over the world on the latest techniques in our specialty, which has been a great privilege. I've lectured to orthodontists in countries such as Russia, Singapore, China, Australia, France, Mexico, Germany, and Italy, just to name a few, as well as most of the states in the United States. I've been able to rub shoulders with some of the best, *and some of the worst*, orthodontists in the world. It's been an amazing ride, and meeting all of these doctors has given me great perspective on the current state of our great profession.

Like many orthodontists, I have spent years in consultations with patients, grabbing those ten- to fifteen-minute windows of time in their lives with both hands, trying desperately to give them the distilled version of what modern orthodontics is, what it may mean to them, and why they've found themselves in a specialist's office.

It's a lot of information, and to be fair, I don't do these patients any favors by rushing through my explanations. This book is an attempt to help demystify the rapidly changing art and science of modern orthodontics for you, the consumer, patient, parent, or individual who may be seeking orthodontic treatment.

My road to becoming an orthodontist was rather circuitous, and I want to share it with you in a nutshell.

I started dental school with the goal of being an oral and maxillofacial surgeon (OMFS). I completed dental school at Baylor College of Dentistry (now Texas A&M University Baylor College of Dentistry) and went on to a residency training program in oral and maxillofacial surgery, the specialty of dentistry that deals with the surgical correction of facial abnormalities, trauma, disease, and the like. The OMFS residency program I attended is based at Parkland Memorial Hospital in Dallas, Texas, the same hospital that President Kennedy was rushed after his assassination.

Parkland has arguably one of the best OMFS programs in the country, and it has produced some of the most renowned surgeons in the field. Medical school at the University of Texas Southwestern Medical School is a part of this training program, and it was a fantastic experience.

As I was nearing completion of my residency program, I realized that although doing surgery was enjoyable, challenging, and fascinating, the lifestyle was anything but. So, with the blessing of my wife, I made a change and completed a two-year residency training program in orthodontics at Eastman

Dental Center at the University of Rochester, in Rochester, New York.

Enough about my background. The truth is that there are a lot of orthodontists out there, all of whom practice the art and science of orthodontics a bit differently. That's great! It's what differentiates one practitioner from another; I prefer to call it style. Style can confuse patients as to what type of orthodontic treatment they should receive or have available to them.

Unlike many specialties in medicine and dentistry, orthodontics is truly both an art and a science, and beauty is in the eye of the beholder. What one orthodontist may consider a successful orthodontic result may not shine so brightly in the eyes of another. I'm just one orthodontist with his own opinion of what makes an attractive smile.

It's with this perspective that I wish to clarify some of the truths of this great specialty. I don't do it because I think I'm the best there is—I'm clearly not—but I am frustrated by the amount of misinformation that is promulgated by dentists and nondentists alike. I hope that, by the end of this small work, you will have a better understanding of what options are available to you and your family members when it comes to considering orthodontic treatment.

Let's get started.

Two

Orthodontics the Way You Remember It (and Would Like to Forget)

I often sit across the consultation table from parents who lament, "When I was a kid, there wasn't a soul that had braces. Anywhere. Kids in grade school just didn't seem to have braces, not until much later in life." I hear that all the time, and guess what? It's true. Kids in first, second, and third grade never seemed to have braces on. Oh, sure, every once in a while some poor sap came to school with braces on the front four teeth— or worse, with headgear—but that was not the norm. Kids just didn't get braces very young, and there was a good reason for it: instead of starting earlier in life with braces to create space for crowded teeth, orthodontists would wait until the child's teen years and extract permanent teeth as a way to create space.

Almost all orthodontists corrected their patients' crowded mouths by removing four permanent teeth in combination with braces. The most common pattern of tooth extraction therapy by orthodontists, but certainly not the only one, was the removal of the upper and lower first bicuspids, or premolars—a procedure also known in orthodontic and surgical circles as "four on the floor." Walk into the oral surgeon's office with crowded teeth, and voila! In less than an hour, there was space in the mouth where before there was none. And, lots of it! Then, over the next two to three years, Megan would go to the orthodontist's office to have her braces tightened as the orthodontist would methodically close the spaces that had been created with extractions.

What we've observed over many years of relying on this relatively easy way to create space is that we've negatively impacted facial profiles. You might have even seen the telltale signs yourself without even realizing it: large nose, thin lips, and large chin. It's a profile alteration that's become so prevalent that orthodontists have a name for it: the extraction profile.

We didn't stop at extractions, either. We did other things that some of us keep locked away in the darker recesses of our memories. How about headgear? It's amazing to me that orthodontists were able to get kids to wear those metal monstrosities to school when I struggle to get kids to wear tiny rubber bands inside their mouths where no one can see them. Kudos to those masters of motivation for getting kids to comply. Maybe kids were just more compliant back then? Whatever the case may be, those devices just aren't necessary anymore. In fact, they can have negative consequences on the facial profile.

Remember palate expanders or splitters? For those of you who didn't have the warm and fuzzy experience of an expander, allow me to paint a picture. Imagine lying on your couch at home while your mom or dad hovered over your open mouth with a "key" that was inserted into a crank cemented to your upper teeth. Every day for several weeks you would have your crank turned with this key.

Often, during this experience, you would have the distinct pleasure of hearing an audible pop, which was the sound of your palate splitting down the middle. It didn't stop at your palate, though; the bone-splitting actually went all the way up to your nasal bones and the bones of your face, separating them from each other. Don't get me wrong: nothing dangerous was happening. In fact, you were doing what the orthodontist wanted: you were splitting your upper jaw in half in an attempt to either get you out of a crossbite, gain room for crowded teeth, or both. Now, if this were the only way to accomplish these goals, then I would have to say "OK, let's do it." It's not, however, and I haven't used an expander to gain space for teeth since I was in my orthodontic graduate residency program.[1]

How about really long treatment times? Remember those days? Perhaps I should say, remember those years? Not so long ago, treatment times of up to four, five, and even six years would be the norm, frequently resulting in permanent tooth damage. However, with the orthodontic techniques available to us today, such long treatment times are simply not necessary. One no longer should expect to find that the removal of their orthodontic brackets might, indeed, reveal a number of unsightly white marks on the teeth where enamel decalcification has resulted from the extended treatment time.

---

[1] That being said, I do think that there is a place for palatal expanders, and that is in young patients who have been diagnosed with airway obstruction. In these children, palatal expansion really can provide relief to breathing difficulties, especially if combined with the removal of large adenoids. We have good evidence to demonstrate that palatal expansion increases the volume of the nasal airway and consequently decreases the resistance to air flow.

Fortunately, through the use of improved treatment techniques, many orthodontists are now able to complete most cases in about half the time it required twenty years ago. Often in a single year, and that's treating *all* of the teeth in the mouth, not just the front teeth.

Needless to say, orthodontics *isn't* the way you remember it, for you or for your child. We've come a long way, baby!

Three

My Dentist or an Orthodontist: What's the Difference?

Relationships are funny things. Sometimes they can cloud our judgment, make us choose irrationality over rationality, and, frankly, keep us from doing the right thing. Just ask any of the many people who are tired of their current hairdresser. Choosing another one can be nearly as difficult as getting a divorce. It's awkward and uncomfortable. Unfortunately the same thing can happen with health care providers. You see it all the time: friends tell you of a great new dentist in town, or a new physician, but you've been with yours for *years*. Let the scheming begin. How are you going to get out of this one?

We should feel lucky when we've got the kind of relationship with our general dentists or primary care dentists (PCDs) that makes us want to stay with them. We trust them. That's fantastic. However, don't let your loyalty guide you down the rosy path that says, "My dentist can do everything." No dentist can—at least not to the level of a specialist. I've seen this assumption—that a general dentist can do everything at the level of a specialist—from a surgeon's perspective and from an orthodontist's perspective.

In dental school, the student is trained to restore and replace teeth damaged by decay and/or periodontal disease. Additionally, each student is exposed to all of the nine specialty disciplines of dentistry, allowing those who wish to pursue a specialty do so by seeking advanced training in a post-graduate specialty program.

The nine dental specialties recognized by the American Dental Association at the time of this writing include:

- Dental public health is the science and art of preventing and controlling dental diseases and promoting dental health through organized community effort.
- Endodontics is the branch of dentistry that is concerned with the morphology,

physiology, and pathology of the human dental pulp and periradicular tissues.

- Oral and maxillofacial pathology is the specialty of dentistry and discipline of pathology that deals with the nature, identification, and management of diseases affecting the oral and maxillofacial regions. It is a science that investigates the causes, processes, and effects of these diseases.

- Oral and maxillofacial radiology is the specialty of dentistry and discipline of radiology concerned with the production and interpretation of images and data produced by all modalities of radiant energy that are used for the diagnosis and management of diseases, disorders, and conditions of the oral and maxillofacial region.

- Oral and maxillofacial surgery is the specialty of dentistry that includes the diagnosis and surgical and adjunctive treatment of diseases, injuries, and defects involving both the functional and aesthetic aspects of the hard and soft tissues of the oral and maxillofacial region.

- Orthodontics and dentofacial orthopedics is the dental specialty that includes the diagnosis, prevention, interception, and correction of malocclusion as well as neuromuscular and skeletal abnormalities of the developing or mature orofacial structures.

- Pediatric dentistry is an age-defined specialty that provides both primary and comprehensive preventive and therapeutic oral health care for infants and children through adolescence, including those with special health care needs.
- Periodontics is that specialty of dentistry which encompasses the prevention, diagnosis, and treatment of diseases of the supporting and surrounding tissues of the teeth or their substitutes and the maintenance of the health, function, and esthetics of these structures and tissues.
- Prosthodontics is the dental specialty pertaining to the diagnosis, treatment planning, rehabilitation, and maintenance of the oral function, comfort, appearance, and health of patients with clinical conditions associated with missing or deficient teeth and/or oral and maxillofacial tissues using biocompatible substitutes.

Now let me be crystal clear: there are PCDs who do provide orthodontic treatment in their offices, and some of them do certain orthodontic procedures quite well. I have absolutely no problem at all if you choose to be treated by your PCD, as long as you are the one who decides to forgo having a specialist do your orthodontics. This is a patient's right-to-know issue, not a dentist's right-to-treat issue. You have a right to know that there are specialists who have thousands of hours of training specifically in one area of dentistry and that general dentists cannot possibly master all specialties or even one specialty without spending the same amount of time that specialists do mastering their craft.

My stepfather-in-law, Don, is a family practice physician who for the first half of his career practiced in the *golden age* of medicine, between the 1950s and 1970s, when patients revered physicians and did just about whatever their primary care providers (PCPs) told them. When Don started his practice in Southern California, he did it all, as many PCPs did. He performed hernia operations, delivered babies, and even performed vasectomies. Yet the time eventually came when he recognized that specialists performed those procedures every day as a matter of routine. It became a moral imperative for Don to hand over the procedures that were best treated by specialists because it was in his patients' best interests. I admire him for that.

In dentistry, as in any profession, there are those practitioners who are scrupulous, like Don, and those who are unscrupulous. When PCDs are scrupulous, when they have done the heavy lifting as far as education, mentorship, and practice are concerned, and when they feel that they can provide their patients the same level of care that a specialist can provide—*and they can explain this to their patients*—then more power to them.

In order to help you understand a bit how an orthodontist is educated, allow me to walk you through an orthodontist's training:

Once accepted into dental school, after completing a four-year college degree with the required hours of science and math, the norm is four years of graduate dental education. In many dental schools, the first year is similar to the first year of medical school, including classes in anatomy, physiology, pathology, biochemistry, pharmacology, etc. Having had the privilege of attending both dental and medical school, I can tell you that the education in that first year is very similar.

Medical and dental schools diverge dramatically, however, starting in the second year. In dental school our second year is focused on the clinical skills involved in dentistry: preparing teeth for fillings, crowns, bridges, and so on. We spend hours in labs hunched over artificial teeth with high-speed drills, learning how to master the subtleties of clinical dentistry. The third and fourth years of dental school are patient focused. During these years, the novice dental students slowly and methodically hone their clinical skills on living patients.

Exposure to specialties in dental school happens in clinics, supervised by either faculty or residents in those particular specialties. As in medical school, these clinical rotations through specialty departments provide young dentists in training exposure to the specialties of their profession. In no way does this brief and very limited time in a specialty clinic provide the training necessary to master any one specialty. This is an introduction, not an education.

Upon entry to dental school, students quickly get a good idea about the specialties available to them. They also gain a quick appreciation for how competitive each of those specialties is and how difficult each is to enter. It is common knowledge in dental school that orthodontics is one of the most competitive residencies available.

This isn't to say that general dentists weren't at the top of their respective classes; they certainly may have been, and they may have chosen general dentistry as their profession.

Once dental students are accepted into a postgraduate orthodontic program, they start an entirely new curriculum. Students complete coursework on growth and development, biomechanics, biology, orthodontic techniques, surgery, TMJ (jaw joint), retention, and other salient topics pertaining to the specialty.

More important, they evaluate, diagnose, and plan treatment for orthodontic patients and then treat those patients and provide them with retainers to preserve the final outcome of their orthodontic treatments. They review hundreds of cases and scour all of the pertinent literature in order to understand the nuances of almost every conceivable orthodontic problem. They then complete rotations through oral surgery, cranio-facial abnormalities, periodontics, prosthodontics, pediatric dentistry, and the like.

Finally, students take part one of the American Board of Orthodontics exam, covering the breadth and depth of the specialty of orthodontics and dentofacial orthopedics. After postgraduate training, they are awarded either a certificate in orthodontics or a master's degree in biology. Then the *real* learning begins.

Jumping into a busy orthodontic practice can be more than daunting. Going from eight to twelve patients a day as a resident to over a hundred patients a day as a busy private practitioner is quite a wakeup call. Yet it's so rewarding and such an education! It is here, in the trenches, day in and day out, that orthodontists master their craft—getting into trouble, getting out of trouble, correcting missteps, and reveling in beautifully treated cases. This is where the learning is!

So, I would suggest that an orthodontic specialist is the best-trained, most expert, and most highly qualified individual to understand the nuances of the art and science of smile enhancement through tooth movement. It's comparing hundreds hours of training that a dedicated PCD interested in orthodontics might participate in with the thousands of hours of combined training and treatment experience that an orthodontist has.

It's why most PCDs have their families treated by orthodontists.

Four

How Do Teeth Move and How Can This Impact the Way We Breathe?

I promise that this chapter will not be an exhaustive essay on the biology and biomechanics of tooth movement. Yet in order to understand the exciting technologies that we have available to us in modern orthodontics, it's helpful to have a very basic understanding of how we move teeth.

The body is dynamic and constantly changing. It responds to environmental stimuli in thousands of ways. The pupils constrict in bright sunlight. The skin releases melanin in response to ultraviolet light. Muscles grow and multiply when challenged with heavy, repetitive movements. Bone changes its shape and density in response to pressure. All of this is the remarkable response of a human organism that is designed not only to react to an external stimulus, but also to adapt to it. Teeth are no different.

When a constant, light pressure is applied to a tooth, it moves. Note that I said *light* pressure. Light pressure is the most efficient way to reshape bone. Keep in mind that when we move teeth, we're really reshaping the bone around the teeth. The teeth are merely acting as a tool to move the bone, or in some instances, to create new bone.

Think of an individual who has scoliosis, a pathological curvature of the spine. For many decades, the way we treated scoliosis was to have the patient wear a back brace that slowly applied corrective pressure to the spine. Over time, the curvature improved. It was far more than just straightening the spine; if you were to observe the shape of each vertebral body, you would notice that it changed over time. It's called remodeling, which is reshaping bone that is already there. But can we actually *grow* bone?

When we have patients with congenital abnormalities that leave them with severely shortened legs, jawbones, or any deficient bones in their bodies, we can lengthen short bones by applying traction to each bony segment. We call this *distraction osteogenesis*, and it's been done for years. It's important to note the roots of the word *osteogenesis. Osteo* means bone, and *genesis* means formation or creation. We create new bone, liver cells, skin cells, and hair cells all the time. The great thing is that we can direct that growth and remodeling; in fact, that's the entire basis of the specialty of orthodontics. Not only can we direct this growth and remodeling, but we're learning how to speed it up! We'll briefly cover that technology in chapter nine.

We didn't always understand how teeth move, even in our very specialized area of orthodontics. The classical theory of tooth movement was that applying lots of pressure to teeth would eventually cause them to move. This is true, but at what cost? We couldn't move them very far, because the body doesn't adapt well to heavy forces. That's why we had to extract teeth so frequently: we just couldn't create the space necessary to accommodate all of the teeth because the body wasn't adapting very efficiently, and it was our fault, because we had the true concept of tooth movement all wrong—and many orthodontists and general dentists still do.

Understanding the correct biology of tooth movement has been quite a revelation for orthodontists. This understanding has allowed us to significantly decrease the number of extractions that we request. In fact, I went back and reviewed the last five hundred consecutive patients I've treated, and my extraction rate was 0.01 percent, a figure that frankly surprised me. Don't misunderstand: there are cases in which permanent tooth extractions are required; however, those should be the exception, certainly not the rule. Avoiding extractions allows us to create broad, beautiful smiles. And that's a great thing.

While we're speaking of permanent tooth extractions, of which you may divine that I'm not a fan, I want to mention another potential downside beyond aesthetics: decreasing the airway.

Let's Take a Breather

It really hasn't been until the advent of three-dimensional cone beam computed tomography (CT) scanning in orthodontics (on which I'll have more to say in chapter eight) that we've really started to see the impact that orthodontists have on the airway—more than ear, nose, and throat (ENT) surgeons and more than sleep specialists. Obstructive sleep apnea (OSA), for instance, is a problem that physicians have known about for years. Mistakenly seen as a problem unique to overweight individuals, OSA is known to increase blood pressure and decrease cognitive performance in individuals of all ages. Left untreated, OSA in its most severe forms is a killer.

I remember reading several research papers during my orthodontic residency that indicated a connection between palatal expanders and the reduction in *nocturnal enuresis* (bedwetting). How weird is that? We put young children in rapid palatal expanders and their bedwetting goes away! It didn't happen every time, but it happened enough for orthodontists to write papers about it. The authors of these studies made casual references to a myriad of plausible explanations, but none of them were very satisfactory.

Now that orthodontists are really starting to grasp our ability to actually change the volume and shape of the nasal passages, floor of the nose, and roof of the mouth—and most important, now that we measure the airway of patients—we are beginning to understand some of the greatest impacts we can have on an orthodontic patient's global health.

I'm willing to bet that the kids whose bedwetting stopped had OSA. Because they didn't sleep well due to constant interruptions from obstructed breathing patterns, they were simply exhausted. When you're so tired you can barely wake up, it's hard to get out of bed when your bladder is full. Correct the breathing issues and allow normal sleep, and the children are rested enough that they do wake up when they sense their bladder is full; thus their bedwetting stops.

I have a personal commitment to evaluating the airway of every child who enters my office. When our daughter was almost four years old, my wife and I decided to have her tonsils and adenoids removed. My wife had noticed how loud her breathing was at night and how grouchy she could be in the morning. We suspected sleep apnea problems and found an understanding ENT surgeon who promptly performed the surgery. Wow, what a difference! Now she sleeps quietly through the night and is a different little girl because she's actually sleeping *well*.

Back to the negative impact of extractions on the airway. Imagine, if you will, having an orthodontist take molds of your upper and lower teeth and then reproduce them in castings of plaster. On those plaster casts, draw an imaginary arc starting from the back molar across the tops of all of the bottom teeth, all the way to the molar on the other side of the mouth. Now picture two of those teeth missing and the spaces closed. Trace the arc across the tops of all the teeth again, and this time it's shorter because two teeth are missing and the space they previously occupied is now gone.

Picture doing that for both the top and bottom teeth. Extracting four permanent teeth results in a reduction in the *volume* of the mouth. This would likely have no impact on your breathing health if you had no tongue. But you *do* have a tongue, and it's got to live in that volume that we just reduced! The tongue moves to the back of the throat, further negatively impacting the airway. Imagine doing this to someone that already has borderline OSA; is it possible that we could make the OSA worse? You bet it is.

OK, Back to How Teeth Move

Constant, low forces move teeth. We know this and we've proven this, yet so many orthodontists and general dentists insist on using high forces. Remember going to the orthodontist and having your braces tightened? Your mouth would hurt for at least a week or more. Then, just as you started to become pain free, you'd go back and the entire nightmare would play itself over, and over, and over. Those were heavy forces that were altogether unnecessary and even harmful in many instances.

This new understanding of tooth movement is also the reason you see children getting braces at younger ages. In fact, the American Association of Orthodontists recommends that all children be evaluated by an orthodontist by the age of seven. Because we know we can create space in young children's jaws, we can jump in early in order to prevent severe crowding in the future. Orthodontists often refer to this early treatment as phase I treatment. Phase I treatment not only takes advantage of light forces generating space for crowded permanent teeth; it also capitalizes on young children's rapid facial growth. Children around the ages of eight, nine, and ten can have short lower jaws redirected such that they can avoid surgery in the future. Even younger children than eight can benefit from appliances, for example, those that help correct underbites.

Phase I treatment doesn't rule out the need for braces when all of the permanent teeth erupt. At that stage we're just getting in and doing the heavy lifting early, so that when all of the permanent teeth erupt into the mouth, we can keep treatment relatively short. We refer to this second part of treatment as phase II. There are plenty of children who don't need phase I; however, only experienced orthodontists taking full advantage of all of the patient's diagnostic records should make the decision as to the need for an early phase of orthodontics.

It's very important to understand that you don't need a general dentist's or pediatric dentist's referral to be evaluated by an orthodontist. You can call and make an appointment for an evaluation for yourself or your child any time you wish, and I really hope you do, for your sake. You see, I've seen literally hundreds of cases where a child *should* have been evaluated by an orthodontist and never was.

So many times I've had to stare awkwardly at a parent who looks me straight in the eye and says, "but why didn't my dentist tell us we needed to see an orthodontist?" I really hate to be the one to tell them that many general dentists either don't know what to look for or just don't notice situations that absolutely beg for orthodontic intervention. Do the right thing and have your children evaluated by an orthodontist by the age of seven.

Many times in that initial consultation with your orthodontist, your child will just be put in growth observation, but sometimes treatment is necessary. The good news is that we've come a long way in our understanding of force management in orthodontics. You will read in chapter six that we now use lighter wires, lighter rubber bands, fewer extractions, less headgear, and gentler visits at the orthodontist's office.

You're welcome.

Five

Why Orthodontics?

A readers' poll in *USA Today* asked 5,500 unat-tached adults age twenty-one and older what qualities they judge most in the opposite sex. They were asked to choose from a list what they look for in an individual they would consider dating—what attributes were the most appeal-ing. Were looks, money, education, family back-ground, or personality traits deciding factors in the choice to date an individual? More precisely, were the choices based solely on appearance? Here are the results:

The top ten characteristics that women use to judge men are
- their teeth (71 percent);
- their grammar (69 percent);
- their clothes (58 percent);
- their hair (53 percent);
- their nails and hands (52 percent);

- their having or not having a tattoo (34 percent);
- their shoes (29 percent);
- the car they drive (24 percent);
- their accent (22 percent); and
- the electronic devices they carry (10 percent).

Electronic devices they carry? Don't ask me.

How about the men?

The top ten characteristics that men use to judge women are
- their teeth (58 percent);
- their grammar (55 percent);
- their hair (51 percent);
- their clothing (45 percent);
- their having or not having a tattoo (40 percent);
- their nails and hands (37 percent);
- their accent (19 percent);
- their shoes (18 percent);
- the car they drive (13 percent); and
- the electronic devices they carry (9 percent).

Of course this wasn't a scientific study by any means, but it does give us a glimpse into the importance of the teeth and the smile. In both sexes, this one variable rose above all others.

We know from well-documented studies that individuals with straight, nice smiles are judged by others to be more intelligent and more successful.

Think about it: a perfect stranger walks up to you looking well dressed and sounding well spoken, but when he opens his mouth, you realize that the gaps between his teeth are so great, or his bite is so bad, he could eat an ear of corn through a picket fence. How we perceive people may be shallow, but sadly, for many, how others are perceived is everything.

It isn't just adults. I can't tell you how many children I've treated who are so self-conscious of their teeth that they can't even smile on command. Smiling spontaneously is totally different from smiling on command. Smiling on command is a learned trait, practiced over and over for taking photographs, feigning happiness, and many other instances where smiling isn't a natural reflex. If you've spent your life consciously keeping people from seeing your teeth because you're embarrassed by them, then it's difficult to smile on command because you haven't practiced it.

I know this because, as a part of the initial records for all of my new patients, I take photos— lots of photos. I take photos of the teeth, yes, but even more important for me, I take facial photos with the patients both in repose and smiling. Most people know how to smile when someone says, "Smile big." Sadly, however, there are many kids (and some adults) who just cannot smile on command. They manage to eke out a crooked worm of a smile that almost looks painful.

Smiles mean so much.

Yet orthodontics isn't only about making beautiful smiles. We orthodontists try very hard to create a harmonious bite that offers the best protection possible against the destructive action of grinding and chewing. We try to minimize the wear that teeth are always subject to in the course of human life. We never stop it completely, but we certainly stem the destruction by properly aligning the teeth.

How about looking more youthful?

Many subtle yet predictable variables conspire to give the face telltale signs of aging, not the least of which is the smile. As we age, our smiles undergo changes as part of a natural course of wear and tear.

We wear down our teeth from grinding, clenching, and chewing. Our upper lips become thinner and start hanging down lower and lower.

This in turn decreases the amount of upper tooth display. Look at the smiles of older individuals compared with their more youthful counterparts: younger people display more of their upper teeth when they speak and when they smile.

As a part of aging, the back teeth tend to tip in toward the tongue. Look at your smile in a mirror right now. If your teeth were like mine before orthodontics, you would note that they do indeed tip inward. The more they tip in toward the tongue, the greater the space between the cheek and the teeth. Dentists call this space the buccal corridor, and we know that the greater the corridor, the less attractive the smile.

Take a look at any *People* magazine. The vast majority of folks in that periodical have spent thousands of dollars in the offices of skilled Beverly Hills general dentists and orthodontists. Look at what they have in common: broad, beautiful smiles. Not only do they have a conspicuous lack of a buccal corridor, but their upper teeth also naturally follow their lower lip line.

That beautiful, youthful sweep of the upper front teeth along the natural curvature of the lower lip is known to orthodontists as the smile arc. The sad part is, there are many orthodontists who don't see and don't appreciate it. I see it all the time as I lecture: instinctively we recognize a beautiful smile, but dissecting it and breaking it down into its constituent parts takes time, work, and experience.

Those dental professionals who recognize these subtle hallmarks of youth have waiting rooms *full* of patients because word gets out on the street that their patients' smiles look different: they look youthful, healthy, and bright. You can't just learn this in a course or even in a full orthodontic residency; it takes spending years with a mentor.

Think about it. If a young, budding artist is enamored with the jaw-dropping blown glass of Dale Chihuly, spending a weekend with him isn't going to do diddly-squat. Spending a *year* with him won't make the young apprentice an artist. It takes years and years of being with and working in the shadow of gifted artists to slowly see what they see and do what they do. That's the whole point of apprenticeship.

I learned very early in my education to model my behavior to mimic those whom I deemed successful: *mentors*. I did it in college, dental school, medical school, surgery residency, orthodontic residency, and most important, *after* my residency, for years.

As a young orthodontist, I started to identify doctors by their completed cases, not by their personalities, education, or monetary success.

I found a couple of gifted orthodontists who consistently produced some of the most beautiful smiles I had ever seen. Their patients' smiles looked youthful, healthy, and *natural*—decidedly not the way my patients looked.

I remember a patient from early in my practice who came to see me several years after I had completed her treatment. She was very upset; she told me that she had just come back from a family reunion and had been relentlessly teased by some of her family members because they said she looked like she had dentures. I was completely mystified. I looked at her initial photos and then back in her mouth—back and forth, back and forth. I didn't get it; her teeth were much straighter than they were before, and her teeth fit together perfectly. Was she crazy? Was I crazy? Nope, neither. I just didn't see what she was trying to articulate, and she couldn't explain it in a manner that could get through my thick skull.

Now I get it.

She was trying to tell this young, thickheaded orthodontist that I had made her smile look manufactured. I had done it just like I was taught in my orthodontic residency: I dutifully placed the brackets where I knew my faculty would have told me to place them, and that was the problem! There was no art, beauty, or youth in her smile; she had no smile arc. Her teeth looked just like the Bonneville Salt Flats just outside of Salt Lake City, Utah: white, straight, and flat. You see, I didn't have the benefit of a mentor at the time. When I look back on our conversation, it makes me sad because I now know what she was desperately trying to communicate.

Not long after the devastating debacle I just described, I identified two orthodontists who were just gifted. They got it. They created such beautiful smiles that I just had to learn to do what they did. It became all-consuming for me. I visited their offices, looked at their cases, and watched them work. Soon, I started teaching with them at the Arthur A. Dugoni School of Dentistry at the University of the Pacific in San Francisco, California. I was there to teach residents how to become orthodontists, but the reality was that I was selfishly learning from these masters. I slowly, over years and years, began to see cases the way they saw them, and most important, to treat cases the way they treated them.

Six

What's New with Braces?

Back in chapter four, I discussed high and low forces moving teeth. Specifically I discussed how lower forces move teeth more efficiently and with less pain and fewer negative effects. How do we actually produce the lighter forces that we know move teeth more efficiently, though? Fortunately, technology is on our side; we've come a long way when it comes to how we manufacture braces and wires.

Back in the day, the only type of braces we had available to us was the type that orthodontists refer to as twin brackets. If you had braces as a child, chances are good that this is the type of orthodontic bracket you had. They were given the moniker of "twin" because of the two sets of wings the bracket used to hold the wire in place. Orthodontists most commonly used little rubber bands, the colors that the patients used to pick out to act as the fastener holding the wires into the bracket. Think about that: every tooth had a tiny rubber band that tightly held the wire in the bracket. That was a lot of friction being generated on the wire, and friction slows everything down in life, including tooth movement. In fact, sometimes friction actually brings tooth movement to a screeching halt.

What if, instead of little rubber bands, we had tiny little doors on the braces that allowed us to lock the wire in but decrease the friction? Well, we have those now; we call them self-ligating braces, and we simply don't need those little elastics anymore. Self-ligation has been a game changer for me and thousands of orthodontists around the world. I now have the ability to gain the precious space I need in crowded mouths without extractions in most cases.

Because of the light, physiologic forces that I'm able to use, I can now do things we never dreamed of a decade ago. When I have a moderately crowded case, or even a severely crowded case in some instances, I don't have to rely on extractions to gain the necessary space. Through gentle adaptation of the jawbones, I am able to reshape the anatomy of the jaws, allowing for all of the teeth to erupt or align into their proper positions. The particular braces that I currently use are called the Damon System, but there are others out there.

I'm certainly not saying that if other orthodontists use another bracket or system then they are behind the times. What I *am* saying is that in a decade, I haven't found a system that does more for me in my hands. It's currently the only way that I would treat my family. All of that being said about the brackets themselves, there are *still* very exciting things happening with regard to the technology of braces:

- *SureSmile* is a system whereby an orthodontist places brackets by hand and inserts wires. Then, after several visits, the orthodontist takes an optical scan by using a special camera on the end of a wand passed over the teeth. A computer renders a three-dimensional representation of the teeth, and the orthodontist adjusts the position of the teeth in the virtual world. A robot—yes, a robot—then bends the wires in the way they need to be bent in order to get the teeth in the position prescribed by the orthodontist.

- *Insignia* is a system that also utilizes high-quality optical scans of the teeth; however, the orthodontist takes the scans prior to placing the braces. The orthodontist then manipulates the teeth virtually on a computer and then mills custom brackets and wires on a case-by-case basis.

- *Incognito* is a system of braces that are placed on the tongue side of the teeth, rendering the orthodontic treatment nearly invisible.

Speaking of invisibility, clear brackets have allowed orthodontists the benefits of wires and braces but with a cosmetic advantage. This, of course, would be meaningless if we still had the metal bands around the teeth that we needed to use in the decades prior to the 1970s. Modern bonding technology has allowed orthodontists the great benefit of bonding the brackets directly to each tooth instead of having a bracket soldered to a band of metal that was cemented around each tooth.

Bonding technology has moved light years beyond the first materials used to bond brackets to teeth. Cosmetic dentistry has been the engine driving this technology, and in my opinion, a tooth should have a band around it extraordinarily rarely and only for very specific reasons. Bands are horrible for hygiene, and they leave little gaps between the teeth when they are removed at the end of a case. Sometimes these little gaps close; other times they don't.

By the way, it's not just the brackets that have changed with technology; the wires have changed too. I'm often asked how those little wires move teeth. The answer lies in their chemistry. Wires can be generally broken down into two camps: adjustable and nonadjustable.

Adjustable wires are just that: wires that can be bent with pliers in the hands of an orthodontist. These wires are typically of two types: stainless steel or an alloy called beta titanium. Nonadjustable wires have the fascinating property of recoil, or springback, which allows them to be deformed when putting them in the brackets, after which the heat inside the mouth returns them to their original shape. Wires like this are made of elements like copper, nickel, titanium, and chromium. Orthodontists will typically work our way through a progression of wires until we get to our final, adjustable wires, at which point we add any necessary bends to optimize the position of the teeth.

Seven

Invisalign

If there is one thing that the makers of Invisalign have done extraordinarily well, it's market their product. I don't recall in the last five to six years ever having met a patient that hasn't at least heard of Invisalign, those clear trays that promise to do orthodontics without brackets and wires. Holy cow, amazing—they really *do* move teeth and really can do orthodontics without braces.

Why don't all patients have Invisalign in their mouths instead of braces then, you ask? Well, not everyone is an appropriate candidate for clear plastic trays as a method of tooth movement. Let's face it: these are plastic trays, not metal wires. There are tooth movements that plastic trays do well, and there are other tooth movements that they struggle with. The key to successful treatment with clear aligners lies in the proper diagnosis, and this takes experience.

Practitioners must fail a lot before they start to observe patterns that allow them to know which cases will predictably treat out well and which will struggle.

Invisalign works like this: The orthodontist takes molds (or digital optical scans) of the upper and lower teeth, along with x-rays and photographs. Those records are submitted to Align Technology, where digital models are made. The technicians at Align then create a setup and send it to the orthodontist or general dentist for approval. Keep in mind that these folks lining the teeth up are not dentists; they are technicians in front of computers, lining up the teeth according to certain parameters that Align has set up for them.

Once the setup is complete, it is critical that the doctor critically review all aspects of the case, including whether the movements represented on the computer screen are even possible. You read correctly: it is often the case that, due to jawbone anatomy, tooth root anatomy, bite interferences, and the like, a setup may arrive on the computer of the treating dentist that will never work in the patient's mouth. The only way to know this is through experience. You can't learn it in a weekend Invisalign course or from watching videos on the Invisalign doctors' website.

Unfortunately, there are many doctors who just accept the treatment plan as outlined by the technician. This translates to treatment that doesn't progress as the computer suggests it will, and everyone gets frustrated. This happens even in experienced hands and often needs to be corrected several times during treatment, through a process called midcourse corrections and refinements.

I said that there is one thing that Invisalign did well and that was marketing. They've actually done another thing very well, and that is confuse the public. You see, in an effort to grow their business, they market themselves heavily both to orthodontists and to general dentists. I don't blame them; I would do the same. However, these general dentists have brochures, window decals, and treatment coordinators who promote the fact that they use Invisalign, further blurring the lines between generalists and specialists in the minds of the public.

You've heard me say this before, and I'll say it again: I have no problem with general dentists doing orthodontics, with Invisalign or braces, as long as they let their patients know that there are specialists who do this and only this every single day of their professional lives.

The fact of the matter is, I love Invisalign; it's impressive technology, and I use it a lot. Remember how I said in the introduction that I've had orthodontic treatment on myself, twice? Well, the first time was with traditional braces, and the second time was with Invisalign. It works, and in the right hands, it works well. The advantages are obvious: You can take them out to eat and to brush and floss. Most people can't tell you're in orthodontic treatment. And they facilitate tooth movement in all directions from the get-go.

There is even an Invisalign product for teenagers conveniently called Invisalign Teen. Ugh! When I first heard this, I couldn't believe it. What a bad idea, right? Give teenagers an orthodontic product they can actually take out of their mouths? Good luck.

Teenagers actually wear their trays extremely well, I've found. I think it's because they realize that their alternative is braces. I make a deal with all of my Invisalign Teen patients that, without any permission from their parents, I reserve the right to throw all of their trays in the trash and slap on braces if I see that they aren't wearing their trays twenty-two hours per day. It seems to work. As an added bonus, Invisalign Teen is a really great option for teens who are active in sports, because they can wear their aligners during practice and games without fear of braces turning their lips into hamburger. Yikes!

The great advantage of using Invisalign as an orthodontist rather than as a PCD is that we can combine treatment methods with the aligners in tricky cases and get some really great results. The other advantage to being an orthodontist is that if things just aren't progressing as planned, we can always fall back on braces if we need to. It's comforting to be in the experienced hands of a specialist, to be sure.

Eight

Lasers and CAT Scans and Screws, Oh My!

Not too long ago, orthodontists had only one tool: braces. When your only tool is a hammer, every problem looks like a nail. You don't even see certain problems if you have no way of fixing them, and there was never a better example of this than orthodontics.

If you had a gummy smile, too bad.

Teeth slanted down to one side, too bad.

Missing teeth, too bad.

You get the picture. We as a specialty were really just a one-trick pony for decades. We could work in concert with other specialists (and still do) in order to achieve excellent outcomes in complex cases, but much of that has changed over the past three to five years. We're talking recent history here!

Miniscrews

In order to understand what miniscrews are, a little background is in order. Orthodontists live in a world of pitting one group of teeth against another group of teeth and pulling or pushing. Picking the correct groups of teeth is a very important exercise because it is what determines which teeth move.

It's a lot like tug-of-war on the beach. Imagine ten people on either side. One side has a 210-pound linebacker as the anchor dude; the other side has me, a robust, 155-pound orthodontist. It's pretty obvious, even if I had the strength of ten men (I only have the strength of three), that it would be challenging against that large anchor. Large teeth generally win against small teeth when pulling on them with braces unless you recruit more small teeth, just as we might win the tug-of-war if we recruited more skinny orthodontists.

However, tie me to a tree, and we can't be beat. Since teeth move—all teeth—it's very advantageous in certain cases to have something in the mouth that doesn't move when we pull on it. We call that *absolute anchorage* because, generally speaking, it really is absolute. What we're talking about are small, sterile bone screws. They are called temporary anchorage devices or TADs for short.

TADs have changed the way we view our challenging cases. There are cases that we would have considered impossible using orthodontics alone only a few years ago, but today they are routine. I love these little screws and the many things that they allow us to do. In fact, when I was an oral surgery resident, I published a scientific paper on the utility of these little screws with jaw fractures.

We used to think that the only way to fix a jaw fracture was with large plates and screws. There actually was a better way, with much smaller screws and little plates, and we demonstrated that on lots of fractures we treated.

When I became a private practitioner in orthodontics, there was a scarcity of these little screws on the market. The screws that were available didn't meet my needs or the needs of many orthodontists, so together with some very smart doctors, I helped create a system of TADs that I and thousands of orthodontists all over the world use to this day. The system is called VectorTAS, and it's manufactured by Ormco, the same company that manufactures the Damon System of braces.

In many cases, I have patients who would ordinarily have to undergo general anesthesia and surgery to correct jaw deformities but who now only need me to place several of these screws so that surgery is altogether avoided.

They really are easy to place, often with only topical anesthetic gel. When I've accomplished all I need to do, they're simply removed and the bone heals quickly and completely.

CAT (CT) Scans

For decades, we orthodontists have utilized two x-rays as a part of our diagnostic records: a side view of the patient's skull, known as a lateral cephalometric head film, and a view of the upper and lower jaws, called a panoramic x-ray. Although these two x-rays were all we had for years and years, they did serve us well.

Enter CT scans, computed tomography to be exact. You are probably familiar with medical CT scans, a technology that delivers a high dose of radiation and then reconstructs multiple slices of the high-resolution images. When I was an intern in general surgery, we ordered abdominal CT scans on nearly all of our patients in the emergency room who complained of abdominal pain.

A few years ago, technology was developed that allowed orthodontists, surgeons, and dentists to get the same type of imaging capabilities with far less radiation and unbelievably detailed imagery. It was truly unlike anything we'd ever seen before. These images can be sliced, diced, rotated, magnified, reconstructed, and even printed by three-dimensional printers. For a time, the radiation that these machines delivered to patients was far less than the amount used in medical CT scans but still more than the amount used in traditional cephalometric and panoramic films.

Enter the machine I currently use, the i-CAT FLX machine. Now I'm able to image all of my patients with crystal-clear, three-dimensional, beautiful, and highly diagnostic scans using less radiation than a single traditional panoramic X-ray. With these incredible images, I'm able to visualize the jaw joints (TMJ), jaws, teeth, sinuses, airway, and many other structures. It's hard for me to remember how I was able to practice without three-dimensional imaging. I and my patients have both benefited from it for over four years now. Needless to say, I'm never going back.

Lasers

As much as I love TADs and CT scans in my practice, little has done more to benefit my patients than the use of diode lasers. We all know about lasers. The word *laser* originated as an acronym for "light amplification by stimulated emission of radiation." The beauty of lasers is that they emit what's known as a coherent beam of light, which differentiates laser light from other light sources. It allows for the light to be exquisitely intense, even to the point of cutting and evaporating tissue, bone, steel, and many other substances.

The wonderful thing about lasers in orthodontics is that they allow us to speed up treatment in some cases. Often, prior to the common use of lasers in orthodontics, we would wait for months and months and months for canine teeth to slowly erupt through the gum tissue. Honestly, we would be done with everything else in the mouth except for those ridiculous canines that were just *bulging* underneath the gum tissue.

If that situation happens today, I simply apply a topical gel anesthetic (no injections), get out my diode laser, and remove the tissue over the tooth, with no pain and no bleeding. No bleeding is key, because it allows me to bond a bracket to the tooth immediately. You see, a tooth needs to be relatively dry in order for the bonding material to adhere the bracket to it. If there is blood in the area, chances are the bonded bracket will fall off soon after it is bonded. Lasers prevent this from happening by keeping the gum tissue from bleeding.

Procedures like this are done all the time in modern orthodontic offices, allowing us to bond braces to teeth much earlier in treatment than we did prior to laser-assisted orthodontics.

Laser-assisted orthodontics doesn't stop at uncovering teeth. Many times I would complete a case and be pretty happy with the result but frustrated that uneven gum tissue around the front teeth was preventing the smile from being all it could be. Now, when a case like this is in my office, I will perform cosmetic gum recontouring of the front teeth after I have completed the orthodontic treatment. It really changes a good case to a fantastic one and a satisfied patient into an incredibly enthusiastic one.

These small adjunctive procedures during and after orthodontic treatment are truly gratifying. Patients' smiles are absolutely stunning—a far cry from when they started treatment. I'm happy, and the patient is happy.

Everyone smiles.

Nine

Accelerated Orthodontics

When adults are asked what's important to them when considering orthodontic treatment, three answers consistently rise to the top: comfort, aesthetics, and time.

In the chapters on braces and Invisalign, I discussed aesthetic advances in modern orthodontics that truly allow the great majority of treatment to go virtually unnoticed. We've gotten much better at addressing the aesthetics concern that adults often share. What has escaped us until now are the other two concerns: pain and long treatment times.

I've long contended that we will never convince the vast majority of adults who would benefit from receiving orthodontic treatment to do so until we get our treatment times close to a year or less. Reducing treatment time has long been a struggle. We've made steps in the right direction by reducing the number of permanent teeth we extract and by capitalizing on low-friction orthodontic techniques, but we still haven't consistently reached the year-in-treatment benchmark. However, we're now getting closer.

Without getting too technical, we are coming to appreciate the fact that tooth movement is largely orchestrated by the same complex cascades of genes, proteins, hormones, and other factors that are also responsible for bone healing. For example, when a bone is fractured, there are multiple genes that switch on and become responsible for triggering an environment of bone remodeling and healing.

One key bone modulating protein is known as RANKL: receptor activator of nuclear factor kappa-β ligand. RANKL is a protein that is encoded by tumor necrosis factor ligand superfamily member 11 (TNFSF11). (I threw that in to impress you.)

If we can stimulate the proteins and genes that are responsible for creating an environment of bone turnover, then we will speed up tooth movement. There are several ways of doing this. The most direct way to effect such stimulation is to create bone trauma. There are procedures that orthodontists can perform to accelerate tooth movement that involve surgically damaging bone by reflecting a flap of gum tissue, by directly visualizing the bone and creating cuts with a surgical instrument, or by using a small screw to perforate through the gum tissue directly into the bone (I know, try not to think too hard about it).

Creating such bone damage has been proven to move teeth more quickly, but the effects don't last forever. The biggest downside of using these methods to accelerate tooth movement is that often we need to reinjure the bone more than once. The phenomenon that allows for rapid tooth movement in the wake of direct bone trauma trails off about six months after the initial surgical procedure, at which point the bone returns to normal.

There are better ways, in my opinion, to stimulate this movement without such trauma. One is for the future and two are in the present.

In the future—and I mean near future, not ten years from now—I really believe that orthodontists will introduce these genes and proteins into the gum tissues locally and trigger faster tooth movement. This type of bone modulation through protein and gene therapy is already proving its efficacy in animal trials. You can be sure that human trials are right around the corner.

Remember lasers? When we last discussed lasers, I mentioned diode lasers for bloodlessly cutting gum tissue. Those lasers are known as contact lasers, so named because nothing really happens unless the tip of the laser actually touches the tissue it is intended to cut. There is another type of laser therapy known as low-level laser therapy (LLLT). It works by aiming laser light at the area of tooth roots, which has been proven to increase tooth movement and decrease orthodontic pain. Studies are already being performed on humans, with very promising results.

Another method that orthodontists like me are currently using to decrease orthodontic pain and increase the speed of tooth movement is micropulse technology. For years, orthopedic surgeons have used micropulse therapy to assist in healing bone fractures that refused to heal, also known as nonunions. Through a device called the Exogen system, orthopedic doctors apply low-intensity, pulsed ultrasound over the area of nonunions, and guess what? The majority of them spontaneously heal without further surgical intervention.

In late 2012, the FDA approved the Acceledent device for orthodontic use, and it's only available by prescription from an orthodontist. Acceledent has a mouthpiece that is custom fitted for a patient who is currently in orthodontic treatment, either with braces or with clear aligner therapy. The patient then turns on the unit, which delivers low-frequency pulses for twenty minutes per day.

The remarkable thing about this technology is that it works! Let me give you a solid example of how much it speeds up treatment time: When you decide you wish to have Invisalign treatment, your doctor will instruct you to wear each set of upper and lower trays for two weeks. At the end of the two-week period, you will open up a new set of trays and start the process over again. If you have twenty-four trays, assuming you had no midcourse corrections or refinements, you would be finished with your treatment in forty-eight weeks, or just under a year. Use your Invisalign with Acceledent, though, and you can change your trays every week instead of every two weeks. You would then complete your orthodontic treatment in only six months! Those are real numbers, and that's a real impact on the length of treatment.

Remember that I stated that the key to being successful with Invisalign treatment is case selection. I now routinely have my patients use Acceledent with their Invisalign treatment, and because I use clinical judgment when diagnosing these patients, I almost never go over a year in their treatments. In fact, most are done in less than six months. Now we're talking!

However, decreased treatment time isn't the only benefit that the Acceledent technology brings to my patients. In fact, if you ask my patients, speed isn't the most important benefit that Acceledent brings to the table; decreased pain is. If I were to try to describe to you the discomfort you can expect to experience upon starting orthodontic treatment, I would try to put it on a scale most of us can relate to. On a scale of one to ten, with one being a hangnail and ten being childbirth, I would say that orthodontic pain can hover around six. That's not insignificant. If you ask patients who use Acceledent where they fall on that scale, though, they will tell you that their pain is somewhere below a one. I know because I ask every single patient, and they all say the same thing. It's truly extraordinary.

Ten

Keeping That Beautiful Smile for Life!

I wish I could conclude this book by saying that after your orthodontic experience, you'll wear retainers for a little while, and then your teeth will remain straight for the rest of your life. If I said that, I would be lying, and if any dental professionals tell you that, they're not being honest with you.

Orthodontists have tried for decades to come up with treatment modalities that will improve what we refer to as stability. *Stability* in the mind of orthodontists can be defined as keeping your teeth in the exact same position as they were the day that the braces or aligners came off.

The research we have in orthodontics tells us that there is no such thing as stability, or at least no stability without the use of retainers. It makes sense: the human body is always changing. Our hair grows; our skin wrinkles and sags; our bones change shape; you get the picture.

What we know is that to keep the teeth beautiful, straight, and unmoved from the day the orthodontic treatment was completed, we must have lifetime retention. Don't get me wrong; there will be the occasional patient who doesn't wear his or her retainers as prescribed and whose teeth will hardly move at all. How do we explain this? Luck.

Expecting to devise a treatment scheme that will guarantee that the teeth won't move after a brief time in retention is an absolute pipe dream. It would be the same as getting a facelift at the age of sixteen and expecting that you would look exactly the same twenty years later. It's preposterous. Keep in mind that the jawbones are living structures; they aren't cement. Bones move in response to pressure (remember the chapter on tooth movement?). Pressure is always present in the mouth, from the cheeks, the tongue, and the grinding pressure from the teeth.

Trust me: wear your retainers for life! In fact, I usually give my patients four sets of retainers. Two retainers are small, flat wires that are bonded to the back of the front teeth, both top and bottom. We call those fixed retainers. The reason for the bonded wires is that the first place noticeable crowding usually returns is in the front of the mouth, most commonly in the lower front teeth. It is really beneficial to have these bonded retainers for life.

In addition to bonded retainers, I will commonly fabricate clear upper and lower retainers that look a lot like Invisalign. They fit right over the bonded retainers. For the first few months after treatment, I ask my patients to wear their clear retainers full time (except for eating and brushing), and then I change them over to nighttime wear, forever. Did you hear me? Forever!

I'll tell you the same thing I tell all of my patients: no matter the type of retainer made for you (different cases require different retention protocols), you must treat them like pajamas for your teeth and never go to sleep without them. Never.

There are advantages to full-coverage, clear retainers over other types of removable retainers: they act as protective covers for your teeth in the face of nighttime grinding, they may help prevent jaw pain, and they hug every tooth. This full coverage prevents teeth from moving in any direction. Wear them, I beg of you!

Well, there you have it. You are now a much better prepared consumer when it comes to orthodontic treatment. You are now far wiser than 90 percent of your friends and family, so share what you've learned with them. Orthodontics is faster, safer, and more comfortable than ever.

I hope you choose wisely and wish you many years of wonderful smiles.

Glossary

I have included terms from the book as well as other terms not found in the book that might help readers in their quest to become more educated about orthodontics.

A

a-lastic ties. Small latex or nonlatex elastic rings used for holding an orthodontic wire into twin brackets or braces.

acid etch. Mild acid used to prepare a tooth surface to more readily adhere to orthodontic adhesive.

activator. See **functional appliance**.

anchorage. Resistance to unwanted tooth movement using a tooth, a group of teeth, or an intraoral or extraoral appliance.

angle classification. Categorization of an individual's bite according to the relationship of the molar and canine teeth.

ankylosis. The fusing of a tooth to the jawbone. A pathologic condition that generally requires surgical removal of the fused tooth.

anterior. Front or forward.

appliance. Anything placed in the mouth, either fixed or removable, that assists in tooth and jaw movement.

arch. Upper or lower jaw.

archform. The general shape of either the upper or lower jaw.

archwire. A metal alloy wire attached to brackets to generate forces that move teeth.

B

band. A metal ring that is placed around a tooth with either a bracket or appliance connected to it.

banding. The act of cementing bands or bonding brackets to the teeth.

bionator. See **functional appliance**.

bonding. See **banding**.

braces. Generic term for small metal or clear appliances that are glued to teeth.

bruxism. Grinding of the upper and lower teeth.

buccal. On the cheek side of the back teeth.

buccal tube. A small metal tube attached to a band or bonded to a tooth to provide a housing for an intraoral or extraoral appliance.

C

c-chain. A stretchable series of connected rings used with braces to move teeth and close spaces.

cephalometric x-ray. Side-view x-ray of the head.

class I bite. A bite that has the proper molar and canine tooth relationship when biting.

class I malocclusion. A bite that has proper molar relationships but has spacing or crowding that prevent some or all of the teeth from meeting properly.

class II bite. A bite in which the upper teeth are too far forward and the lower teeth are too far back when biting.

class III bite. A bite just opposite class II, in which the upper teeth are too far back and the lower teeth are too far forward.

crossbite. A bite in which any of the upper teeth are inside the lower teeth when biting.

crowding. A spacing issue in which the upper or lower teeth don't have enough room to erupt into the mouth straight and harmoniously.

D

DDS/DMD. Doctor of Dental Surgery and Doctor of Dental Medicine, respectively. Equivalent degrees. Yes, they mean the same thing. All orthodontists educated in North America will have the abbreviation of one of these degrees after their names, plus an additional two to three years of specialty training beyond their dental degree.

debanding/debonding. The removing of orthodontic appliances.

deep bite. A bite in which the upper front teeth cover or nearly cover the lower front teeth.

dentition. The teeth.

diode laser. A contact laser that removes gum tissue either for facilitated tooth movement or cosmetics.

E

e space. The difference in size between the primary second molar and the permanent second bicuspid. Since the second bicuspid is generally smaller than the primary second molar, there is additional space available upon permanent tooth eruption.

ectopic eruption. A condition in which a tooth erupts into an improper location or position in the mouth.

elastics. Small rubber bands used during orthodontic treatment to move groups of teeth. These may be latex or nonlatex based.

eruption. The growth of the teeth into the mouth.

expander. Any appliance used to expand either the upper or lower jaw.

extraction. Removal of a tooth or teeth.

F

facemask/facebow. An appliance, used outside of the mouth, that attaches to appliances inside the mouth to facilitate forward movement of the upper jaw and teeth while restricting the forward growth of the lower jaw.

fiberotomy. A surgical procedure to sever fibers of the tooth socket around the neck of a tooth. Usually used in an attempt to decrease postorthodontic relapse or movement.

fixed appliances. A common way of describing braces that are glued or otherwise attached to the teeth.

frenectomy. The surgical release of a band of tissue (frenum) associated with either the lip or the tongue.

functional appliance. One of a number of appliances that, when inserted in the mouth, causes the jaws to move into a desirable relationship. Can be either fixed (cemented) or removable and is removed when the desired relationship between the jaw and the teeth is achieved.

G

gingiva. Gum tissue.

gummy smile. A smile that displays a large amount of gum tissue. May have several different causes.

H

happy. What you will be after you complete your orthodontic treatment.

headgear. An appliance, used outside of the mouth, that attaches to appliances inside the mouth. Used to retract the position of the upper jaw and teeth.

Herbst appliance. See **functional appliance**.

I

impaction. A tooth that doesn't erupt into the mouth when expected.

impressions. Using a gelatinous substance to capture the shape of the teeth either to have models made for study or for appliance fabrication.

interceptive orthodontics. Phase I orthodontic treatment.

interproximal reduction (IPR). Removal of small amounts of enamel, either to facilitate tooth movement or to improve aesthetics.

L

labial. On the surface of the front teeth that faces the lips.

ligation. The act of holding a wire against the brackets.

ligatures. Either small elastic rings or segments of wire used to hold the archwire into the brackets.

lingual. On the tongue side of the teeth.

lip bumper. An appliance attached to molars that uses lip forces to move posterior teeth in a backward direction.

M

malocclusion. A condition in which the teeth do not fit together properly.

mandible. Lower jaw.

maxilla. Upper jaw.

mixed dentition. The developmental stage in children in which there is a combination of primary and permanent teeth in the mouth.

mouthguard. An appliance designed to protect the teeth and lips during athletic activities.

N

Nance holding arch. A retainer designed to hold upper molars in position until all permanent teeth have erupted.

nightguard. An appliance worn during sleep, designed to decrease the negative effects of grinding.

O

open bite. A malocclusion in which the upper and lower teeth do not overlap, allowing the tongue to rest on the teeth when the jaws are closed.

orthodontics and dentofacial orthopedics. The dental specialty that includes the diagnosis, prevention, interception, and correction of malocclusion, aesthetic smile design, and the improvement of neuromuscular and skeletal abnormalities of the developing or mature orofacial structures.

P

palatal expander. A fixed or removable device used to expand the upper jaw. See also **expander**.

panoramic x-ray. An x-ray that rotates around the patient's head and captures a two-dimensional image of the jaws, jaw joints, and teeth.

plaque. A colorless, sticky film of bacteria, food, and saliva that constantly forms on the teeth. Plaque combines with sugar to form an acid that damages teeth and gums. Plaque is responsible for tooth decay and gum disease.

posterior. Back or rearward.

primary care dentist (PCD). A general dentist.

R

retainer. Any appliance worn in the mouth to prevent teeth from moving.

rubber bands. See **elastics**.

S

separator. An elastic o-ring or small wire loop placed between the teeth to create space for the placement of bands.

serial extraction. Extraction of certain primary teeth or permanent teeth over a period of time to create room for permanent teeth.

space maintainer or spacer. An appliance, usually fixed, intended to hold space in the mouth to allow for the eruption of permanent teeth.

supernumerary tooth. An extra tooth that generally needs to be removed.

T

tongue thrust. Abnormal positioning of the tongue behind the teeth during swallowing. Forces generated by the tongue can move the teeth and bone and may lead to an anterior or posterior open bite.

T-Rex. A common type of palatal expander that combines expansion with the distalization (rearward positioning) of the maxillary molars.

About the Author

Dr. John Graham received his bachelor of science degree from Brigham Young University. He received his dental degree from Baylor College of Dentistry in Dallas, Texas, and then received his medical degree from the University of Texas Southwestern Medical School. After medical school, Dr. Graham completed an internship in general surgery at Parkland Memorial Hospital, followed by training in oral and maxillofacial surgery.

Following his surgical training, Dr. Graham received his certificate in orthodontics from the University of Rochester/Eastman Dental Center in Rochester, New York. Dr. Graham is one of only a handful of orthodontists in the United States who are also physicians.

An innovator, educator, and in-demand lecturer, Dr. Graham gives presentations worldwide to both doctors and orthodontic staff on the most advanced orthodontic treatment approaches available. Dr. Graham has several patents pending and has been awarded a US patent for an orthodontic device.

He has coauthored multiple orthodontic textbook chapters and has written many professional journal articles. Dr. Graham holds faculty appointments at the University of the Pacific, the Arthur A. Dugoni School of Dentistry, and the University of Rochester's Eastman Institute for Oral Health. Dr. Graham is a contributing editor for the *Journal of Clinical Orthodontics* and *Orthotown* and a reviewer for *Orthodontics: The Art and Practice of Dentofacial Enhancement.*

Dr. Graham is a past president of the Arizona State Orthodontic Association and a member of the Utah Dental Association, the American Association of Orthodontists, the Salt Lake District Dental Society, and the Rocky Mountain Society of Orthodontists.

Dr. Graham and his wife, Dr. Debbie Graham, live in the heart of Salt Lake City, Utah, and, along with their four children, love to ski, bike, attend sporting events, and spend quality time together.

Made in the USA
Middletown, DE
16 August 2016